Distribution, publication, and copying in any form are prohibited and subject to damages.

TEN HYPNOSES

Copying, publishing, and sharing with third parties are only permitted with the written consent of the author. Please observe the notes on copyright and usage.

Distribution, publication, and copying in any form are prohibited and subject to damages.

Copying, publishing, and sharing with third parties are only permitted with the written consent of the author. Please observe the notes on copyright and usage.

Distribution, publication, and copying in any form are prohibited and subject to damages.

Ingo Michael Simon

TEN HYPNOSES

24
FEELINGS OF GUILT

Copying, publishing, and sharing with third parties are only permitted with the written consent of the author. Please observe the notes on copyright and usage.

Distribution, publication, and copying in any form are prohibited and subject to damages.

© 2024 Ingo Michael Simon
All rights reserved.
Independently published
www.ingosimon.com

Important Notes for Urgent Attention:
The contents of this book are based on the practical experiences of the author with hypnosis applications and psychotherapy in a trance state. Although the author has strived for the utmost care, errors or misunderstandings in the presentation cannot be completely excluded. Therapeutic work with people and the application of hypnosis are solely the responsibility of the hypnotist. It cannot be ruled out that parts of this book may be misunderstood or that the application of a presented procedure may cause an undesirable reaction in the client. The author also assumes no co-responsibility if work with a client is carried out with reference to the statements in this book.

The Author:
Ingo Michael Simon studied psychology and education and is a hypnotherapist with practices in southwestern Germany and Switzerland. With the help of hypnosis-supported psychotherapy, he primarily treats people with persistent psychological conditions. His practice focuses on anxiety disorders, pathological compulsions, and psychosomatic illnesses. His therapeutic offerings mainly include classical and modern hypnosis applications and the dreamland therapy he developed himself.

Copying, publishing, and sharing with third parties are only permitted with the written consent of the author. Please observe the notes on copyright and usage.

Notes on Copyright and Usage

Copying, publishing, and sharing with third parties is prohibited and only permitted with the written consent of the author. Please observe the following copyright and usage guidelines.

This work has been carefully crafted and created to the best of the author's knowledge and personal experience. It comprises text templates and application guidelines for professional hypnosis sessions. The author is a licensed psychotherapist with extensive experience in psychotherapy, coaching, and personal training using hypnotic techniques and methods. Nevertheless, the author and the publisher assume no liability for the accuracy of information, instructions, and advice, nor for any typographical errors. The author and publisher accept no responsibility or liability for the application of these texts and recommendations with clients or patients, nor for any potential consequences or unexpected reactions. It is expressly noted that the application of therapeutic and advisory techniques and formulations lies solely and entirely within the responsibility of the practitioner. This also applies to adherence to the boundaries of legally regulated medical and therapeutic practices. The fact that a book containing action proposals is freely available for sale does not imply that its application with clients or patients is permitted for everyone.

Distribution, publication, and copying in any form are prohibited and subject to damages.

Copying, publishing, and sharing with third parties are only permitted with the written consent of the author. Please observe the notes on copyright and usage.

Distribution, publication, and copying in any form are prohibited and subject to damages.

Table of Contents

Introduction 9
Hypnosis 1 11
Hypnosis 2 16
Hypnosis 3 21
Hypnosis 4 26
Hypnosis 5 31
Hypnosis 6 36
Hypnosis 7 40
Hypnosis 8 45
Hypnosis 9 51
Hypnosis 10 56
Overview of All Titles in the Series "Ten Hypnoses" 61

Copying, publishing, and sharing with third parties are only permitted with the written consent of the author. Please observe the notes on copyright and usage.

Distribution, publication, and copying in any form are prohibited and subject to damages.

Copying, publishing, and sharing with third parties are only permitted with the written consent of the author. Please observe the notes on copyright and usage.

Introduction

The series "Ten Hypnoses" is very well known in Germany, Austria, and Switzerland as a collection of texts for therapeutic work and is used by numerous psychotherapeutic practices, doctors, therapists, coaches, and other helping professionals. I am pleased to now be able to offer these texts in other countries as well.

Most therapists have their own methods for inducing and deepening trance as well as for exiting trance. Therefore, I have focused on the main part of the hypnosis. The texts in this book can be integrated as the main part into any hypnosis process.

The texts in this collection use various hypnosis techniques. I will not explain these in detail, as I assume that users have the appropriate training. It is also not necessary to understand the exact structure or functioning of the different parts. The texts can simply be read aloud, and they will have their effect.

Decide for yourself which text best suits your client or patient at any given time. You can also combine passages from different texts. It is not about using all ten hypnoses in sequence. It is a selection of possibilities.

I want to emphasize that books cannot replace therapy. Psychotherapy or other therapeutic treatments involve much more. A careful diagnosis is the necessary basis for deciding on the use of methods, including whether hypnosis or one of my texts should be used. Even in this case, preparatory discussions, follow-up discussions during the session, and of course, a therapeutic concept for the sequence of sessions and the content approaches are essential parts of therapy. This cannot and should not be achieved with a collection of texts.

In any case, I wish you much success in your work and I am pleased if my text templates can contribute in a small way.

Ingo Michael Simon

Hypnosis 1

Goal Setting and Strengthening of Will

You have decided to let go of your feelings of guilt... ... So many things you felt guilty about in your life were never your responsibility... ... Often you felt a bad conscience without really being guilty or able to change anything... ... But you no longer want to be guilty... ... You want to shed the burden of these feelings... ... even if your mind is convinced of guilt, you cannot change the past... ... Guilt feelings only hold you back... ... But you want to be free... ... You want to turn to life with a good feeling and enjoy it... ... You want to take care of yourself and not always think about others... ... You may be the most important person in your life... ... Who could be more important in your life than yourself... ... You want and can let go of feelings of guilt and be free again... ... You are determined to achieve this today... ... to take a big step today and already let go of a large part of the feelings of guilt... ... It is truly amazing how well this can succeed once this decision is firmly made... ... and your decision is made...

Thought Alignment

It was your thoughts that often blocked you; now it is this special thought that frees you... ... this one thought that tells you... ... I let go of feelings of guilt because I don't need them anymore at all... ... and every time you consciously formulate this thought, when you think it, it feels right and good... ... I let go of feelings of guilt because I don't need them anymore at all... ... This is the thought of the present... ... it is the thought that counts because all thoughts of guilt belong to the past... ... are over... ... It is a thought that guides and carries you... ... and this thought also helps you feel naturally free and well... ... I let go of feelings of guilt because I don't need them anymore at all... ... This is your guiding thought...

Somatic Alignment (Body Suggestion)

Right now, you are feeling a state of physical calm that is also a state of emotional inner peace, and you are becoming fully aware of this feeling... ... You feel inside and can sense this pleasant and warm relaxation you are in now... ... This calm that also allows you to simply let your feelings be and become freer and more accepting of yourself in deeper relaxation... ... just as you are... ... because feelings of guilt dissolve and are replaced by self-love... ... Your body helps you with this, showing you with its relaxation that the process of becoming free works, that you can actually let go of feelings of guilt and thus feel freer... ... because letting go of guilt means becoming free and becoming one with your own feelings... ... exactly this is what you are achieving and you can trace and feel it in the relaxation of your body... ... You can feel it... ... the peace and relaxation of your body at this moment helps you with this...

Emotional Alignment (Feeling Suggestion)

You look even deeper into your feelings and are fully immersed in your emotions... ... in your inner center where all your feelings reside... ... and right now a completely new feeling is growing there... ... the feeling of freedom... ... initially as a feeling that you have somehow become lighter... ... as if shackles were loosened and you can breathe freely again... ... with each breath, this feeling becomes more beautiful and intense... ... with each breath, you feel that you can breathe more freely... ... breathe more freely because you are getting air deep in your soul again...

... freed from guilt, you can breathe deeply... ... maybe you can feel it clearly already at this moment, or you will feel it even more clearly in a few moments... ... after a few breaths... ... You can manage to free yourself from guilt over and over again... ... you can do it here and now... ... at this moment... ... Now... ... You feel inner freedom and self-love... ... Now...

Behavioral Alignment

You are now also changing how you treat yourself... ... You are determined to consciously feel your inner freedom and experience it over and over again, knowing that it is there and will grow even more... ... You resolve to take better care of yourself... ... to pay more attention to your feelings and feel what you truly feel... ... to feel freedom and self-love... ... as much as possible... ... You are determined to spend moments of reflection fully with yourself... ... fully in your feelings... ... and with deep breaths, feel your inner freedom because only those who are free inside can truly breathe deeply in and out... ... and you can do that now... ... Feelings of guilt are far away... ... Freedom is very near...

Outlook and Vision

You imagine how this will change your life today and tomorrow... ... how inner freedom makes everyday life so much easier... ... You visualize in your mind's eye, in pictures and thoughts, how it will be when you go through the day with this new feeling of life... ... You imagine how you manage to do what is important and good for you and feel good about it... ... completely free of guilt and full of freedom and lightness... ... because you increasingly trust that your deep feelings can be free from bad conscience and guilt and can remain free... ... You will no longer relinquish the decisions of your life... ... you will align your decisions according to your feeling about yourself... ... You will decide for yourself because you know that you can rely on yourself and your feelings...

Summary

It's time, and now there is no other way but to put yourself at the center of your life... ... Liberation from feelings of guilt means becoming free for yourself and first and foremost taking care of yourself and your feelings... ... I let go of feelings of guilt because I don't need them anymore at all... ... This thought is now your most important thought... ... With this thought that imprints itself into your body feeling and thus becomes a matter of course, you begin each new day... ... I let go of feelings of guilt because I don't need them anymore at all...

Hypnosis 2

Goal Setting and Motivation

...... Everything is good now, and you can just let yourself fall into the calm of trance...... and thus you achieve a deep and liberating trance......

...... Everything is good now, and you can just let yourself fall into the calm of trance...... and thus you come closer to yourself today than ever before......

...... Everything is good now, and you can just let yourself fall into the calm of trance...... and thus you become open and ready for a new and conscious path......

...... Everything is good now, and you can just let yourself fall into the calm of trance...... and in peace, you can let all the words take deep and liberating effect......

Thought Alignment

...... Now you can also let go of all thoughts of guilt, just let them drift away...... and feel the inner freedom and peace you are experiencing now......

… … Now you can also let go of all thoughts of guilt, just let them drift away… … and thus you create space for new thoughts and feelings… …

… … Now you can also let go of all thoughts of guilt, just let them drift away… … and thus you internally prepare for self-forgiveness and letting go… …

… … Now you can also let go of all thoughts of guilt, just let them drift away… … and let all the helping words find their way deep inside… …

Somatic Alignment

… … Just be here and perceive your body feeling of relaxation… … and in your body feeling, you feel deep connection with yourself… …

… … Just be here and perceive your body feeling of relaxation… … and in this body feeling, forgiveness and reconciliation from you for you arise by themselves… …

… … Just be here and perceive your body feeling of relaxation… … and in this body feeling, a new and free feeling of life begins… …

… … Just be here and perceive your body feeling of relaxation… … and in this body feeling, feelings of guilt truly dissolve… …

Emotional Alignment

… … Let your new feelings arise and accept them, for they belong to you… … and you recognize that there are many beautiful and free feelings within you… …

… … Let your new feelings arise and accept them, for they belong to you… … and you recognize that accepting these feelings makes you freer and lighter… …

… … Let your new feelings arise and accept them, for they belong to you… … and you recognize that there are more feelings of freedom within you than you thought… …

… … Let your new feelings arise and accept them, for they belong to you… … and you recognize that feelings of guilt and a bad conscience now disappear… …

Behavioral Alignment

… … You can now set a new goal for yourself because you will achieve your goal… … your goal of freeing yourself from harsh self-criticism and self-condemnation… …

...... You can now set a new goal for yourself because you will achieve your goal...... your goal of self-respect and self-recognition......

...... You can now set a new goal for yourself because you will achieve your goal...... your goal of self-acceptance and self-love......

...... You can now set a new goal for yourself because you will achieve your goal...... your goal of a new and free life......

Consolidation

...... Now you can linger in the calm of the liberating trance and simply enjoy the relaxation because everything new begins in calm...... and thus your new life begins in this trance, free from old and exaggerated feelings of guilt......

...... Now you can linger in the calm of the liberating trance and simply enjoy the relaxation because everything new begins in calm...... and thus you also feel new trust in life and especially in yourself......

...... Now you can linger in the calm of the liberating trance and simply enjoy the relaxation because everything new begins in calm... ... You feel the change... ... You feel the liberation and renewal... ... You feel your new and free feelings... ... You feel your new and confident life... ...

Hypnosis 3

Anchor Technique (Post-Hypnotic Anchor)

An anchor (or trigger) is a stimulus that is supposed to create a specific feeling or evoke a particular thought. It is a signal that the client perceives and then initiates an internal process. The established anchor then replaces the suggestion. In everyday life, a client can use an anchor to trigger or create a desired state, even without being in a trance state. Numerous stimuli can be used as anchors/triggers. I work with the following options, which I also use in the series "Ten Hypnoses": Body anchors (closing the hand, pressing the thumb pad...), visual anchors (symbols, word cards...), acoustic anchors (signal sounds like phone rings, melodies...), olfactory anchors (scent oils...), haptic anchors (hand comforters, talismans...). I also differentiate between peri-hypnotic and post-hypnotic anchors. Peri-hypnotic anchors are those mainly used during hypnosis, where the therapist sets the anchor and then repeatedly triggers it as a supplement to suggestions and visualizations. Post-hypnotic anchors are mainly set up for the time after the session, so the client can help themselves with them.

Preparation of the Anchor Technique

Today we are working with an anchor... ... with a small aid that makes it easy for you to focus on yourself and the responsibility you truly have... ... the responsibility for yourself... ... too often you have borne responsibility for others, even when you were not actually responsible... ... and so you have often felt guilty when others suffered or were sad because something was missing or something did not work out... ... but you were not responsible... ... and you have decided to take responsibility for yourself first and foremost from now on, to take care of yourself... ... and not to take on the worries of others as your own guilt... ... You have this thought, this intention that tells you... ... I am primarily responsible for myself... ... You want to firmly anchor this thought to avoid falling into the trap of guilt when you cannot solve another person's problems...

[Prepare a card with the inscription "I am primarily responsible for myself" and discuss before the hypnosis that you will give the client the card during the session. They do not need to open their eyes for this. Announce a touch once more just before handing over the card and touch the client's hand with it so they can grasp it. Follow the instructions in the text!]...

Creating the Desired Emotional State

First, it is all about a beautiful calm... ... because deep in calm and relaxation, it is much easier to let go of disturbing feelings of old guilt... ... and then build a feeling of inner freedom... ... and this feeling of freedom arises when you focus more on yourself... ... bear your responsibility... ... the responsibility for yourself... ... and that means taking care of yourself... ... to then be there for others without guilt or bad conscience... ... who still bear their own responsibility... ... Now you feel the relaxation... ... and in the state of relaxation, you also feel free from guilt... ... very light inside... ... the more you succeed in focusing on yourself at this moment... ... in exactly this moment... ... the better you can now feel inner lightness... ... inner lightness and freedom... ... Now you don't have to take care of anything... ... now you don't have to be there for anyone... ... now you have calm...

Setting the Anchor

Now in the pleasant relaxation, you can meet yourself without judgment, let go of all self-accusations, and accept yourself... ... It works much better now than before... ... You accept yourself at this moment and are free from guilt... ... The more clearly you can feel the relaxation now, the better you can accept yourself without judgment... ... Feel the relaxation and accept yourself without judgment... ... Now... ... Now it works... ... You can feel calm and accept yourself without judgment... ... Now I am giving you the card in your hand... ... [Touch the client's hand and hand them the card. They can keep their eyes closed.] ... ... Feel the card in your hand... ... You know what it says... ... it says: I am primarily responsible for myself... ... You think about this sentence, this attitude... ... You feel that you are not responsible for everyone else... ... You recognize that you often felt guilty because you thought you should have done more for others or taken better care of them... ... Now, however, you focus on yourself... ... resolve to take responsibility for yourself as it says on the card and thus take good care of yourself... ... not to let guilt arise that has nothing to do with you... ... that can have nothing to do with you... ... The card reminds you of this and helps you because whenever you carry it with you, you automatically pay attention to not taking on others' responsibility... ... You succeed... ... you succeed excellently... ... You know that you often learned feelings of guilt and that they were not your true feelings... ... You can free yourself from them over and over again... ... just like today... ... the card helps you with this...

Consolidation (Post-Hypnotic Suggestion)

You can carry the card with you every day... ... and whenever you feel that feelings of guilt are catching up or trapping you, even though you are not responsible for what is happening... ... you can hold it in your hand and read what it says... ... I am primarily responsible for myself... ... and immediately you feel deeper calm and the feeling of freedom inside... ... just like now... ... exactly like now... ... with just one look at the card... ... even when you hold the card in your hand or touch it without reading it, you feel the liberation from feelings of guilt... ... just like today... ... every day, exactly like today...

Hypnosis 4

Preparation and Strengthening of Will

Self-reproach and feelings of guilt have plagued you for a long time... ... You know you cannot change the past, no one can... ... Guilt feelings block you, stand in your way... ... You know they were exaggerated, that you have the right to feel free again... ... To do this, it is important to change your attitude towards yourself... ... the mind can do this quickly, but today it should also succeed in your feelings... ... Today you can experience the feeling of inner freedom... ... experience and consolidate it... ... affirm it, which means making it firm...

Distancing Active Thoughts

Deep inside you, there is a place of clarity... ... At this place, there is only white, pure light... ... You stand at this place and see light all around you... ... Let this image become very clear... ... white light all around you... ... only light everywhere... ... Dive completely into the image of pure white light and perfect inner freedom... ... The ground beneath your feet seems glassy... ... you can see through it... ... infinitely far into the depth... ... But even there you only see pleasant, white light... ... You look up and see light above you too... ... It is everywhere... ... bright and clear and very pleasant... ... It envelops you and gives you clarity and openness... ... You see a glass wall in front of you... ... You can look through it and see only light behind the wall... ... It is beautiful at the place of clarity... ... so pure... ... so free... ... so bright and clear... ... so distinct...

Presentation of the Affirmation

You look at the wall in front of you again... ... Slowly, writing appears in thick, clear letters, becoming more and more distinct... ... You can recognize the writing... ... You can clearly read it... ... On the glass wall in front of you, at the place of clarity, it says...

I let go of all feelings of guilt because they are outdated, I may and can and want to feel free.

... [Read the affirmation slowly and slightly louder than the previous text to emphasize it a bit. Then pause for about 30 seconds before continuing to read.] ...

Impact and Deepening of the Affirmation

Let the words simply flow into you... Let them unfold their effect and give yourself calm and mindfulness... Calm and mindfulness... Embrace yourself inwardly and feel the effect of the words you can read on the glass wall in front of you... ... because everything you take in during a state of inner relaxation, in a beautiful trance, can unfold deeply within you... ... if it aligns with your wish and goal... ... and you have exactly this wish... ... to be free and stay free... ... feelings of guilt that once were there but are long outdated, to let go of... ... because deep inside, you know they cannot help you... ... that they are no longer justified... ... maybe never were... ... Perhaps you can already feel the inner lightness spreading and permeating your emotions... ... or you will feel it even more clearly in a few minutes when the affirmation unfolds even more... ... because it will... ... It unfolds and becomes stronger until it has become your stable belief... ... your new stance of inner freedom... ... freedom from guilt and bad conscience, for both are outdated... ... once they served a function for you, but are no longer significant... ... what matters now is the feeling of freedom and lightness...

Repetition and Integration of the Affirmation

Deep inside, the words echo that you have read and can look at again and take in once more...

I let go of all feelings of guilt because they are outdated, I may and can and want to feel free.

... ... and now enjoy the calm you are in... ... it is truly astonishing how well you can feel calm with these words... ... calm that shows you that you have indeed let go of feelings of guilt now... ... and can let go of them again and again... ... That is right and good... ... that is very good... ... You succeed at this moment in taking in the significance of these words and making them a new and lasting belief... ... your liberation affirmation...

Consolidation (Post-Hypnotic Suggestion)

Very good... ... You have already done everything you need to... ... have changed your belief... ... have taken in a new and correct belief as an affirmation and deeply internalized it... ... and as an affirmation, as a consolidation of your correct belief... ... your correct and constructive new stance towards yourself, you can use this affirmation every day... ... start each day with it and look in the mirror in the morning, just like today at the glass wall... ... and say:

> I let go of all feelings of guilt because they are outdated, I may and can and want to feel free.

... ... So your mirror becomes the glass wall at the place of clarity, and you can stand at the place of clarity every day and say your affirmation... ... can write it on the mirror if you want... ... Every day you begin with a walk to the place of clarity in your home and can read the words on the glass wall and most importantly feel them deeply inside... ... and free yourself again and again... ... until you feel really free and well... ... every day...

Hypnosis 5

Goal Setting and Preparation

You have realized that there are old feelings of guilt within you that do not belong to you... ... You only took them on because no one else was there to bear the responsibility... ... or because you were used to always taking responsibility... ... and with the responsibility can come the feeling of guilt when something did not succeed... ... when something broke... ... when something ended... ... But you have also realized that it is time to let go of old and not truly belonging feelings of guilt... ... You have tried, and sometimes it worked, but somehow a part of the feelings of guilt often remained... ... but today you want to let go of the guilt once more... ... to let go once and for all, because it is time to do so now... ... It is time... ... today you let go...

Perspective Change

Imagine you could place your feelings of guilt next to you... ... could just set them aside and look at them from the outside... ... and then change them... ... maybe just leave them like a heavy backpack that you simply no longer want to carry... ... or smash or grind them into dust... ... maybe then you could always dissolve the feelings of guilt... ... would stand still to dispose of them because you would know that it is indeed possible... ... then it would always become light inside you... ... You could always find new strength... ... could recover and always come back to a good feeling... ... could break down guilt... ... always...

Reevaluation of Own Experiences

You now dive once more into your memories and think of a situation where you felt particularly guilty... ... or a situation or event that made you feel guilty afterward... ... Imagine the opportunity now once more and imagine you placed the guilt like a heavy stone beside you... ... with all the burden that guilt means... ... you could have freed yourself... ... Imagine, with your thoughts, you could have let the stone crumble to dust... ... But you carried the guilt like stones with you, had no hand free to act... ... you had to always carry new stones and balance them... ... You thought you had to bear this burden... ... and whenever you tried to put it down, you later picked it up again and continued to carry it... ... even though you had already put it down... ...

today you know you don't have to carry it anymore... ... and you don't want to carry it anymore... ... Now imagine you place the stones of guilt, the burdens you carried for so long, on the ground... ... You look at them and it is a big pile of stones... ... too big to carry them all... ... You now feel the relaxation, now you feel freer than before... ... and you concentrate on your breath... ... like the wind of time, your breath passes over the stones and dissolves them before your eyes... ... they crumble to dust... ... first, they slowly crumble apart... ... pieces of the guilt stones fall to the ground... ... then they crumble to dust before your inner eye... ... The more you can focus on the thought that your inner peace grows with each breath, the faster the stones of guilt disintegrate within you... ... You see this image before you and let it become clearer... ... Guilt disintegrates into dust... ... Guilt disintegrates into dust...

Action Change

Imagine you would feel guilty in the future... ... would feel that a bad conscience is burdening you... ... and then you act... ... then you place the guilt like a heavy stone next to you... ... make it clear to yourself that holding on to guilt holds you back... ... that feelings of guilt only slow you down and that you can never change the past because it has already happened... ... also, what makes you feel guilty, you can no longer change because it is always events or actions that lie in the past... ... But you can let go... ... you can hand over the old guilt to the past... ... just as the wind wears away every stone over time and returns it to the earth as dust... ... so you hand over feelings of guilt to the past... ... let them be in the place of memory, but not in the present... ... Guilt disintegrates into dust, because then you can best learn from actions and events and change the present... ... Guilt disintegrates into dust... ... like stones in the wind... ... Now you can imagine it before your inner eye, and in a few moments, all the stones of guilt will disintegrate... ... always...

Consolidation (Post-Hypnotic Suggestion)

You now feel the inner calm and relaxation... ... You feel and you know that you can let go of feelings of guilt like stones... ... what once seemed impossible to you is now possible... ... because it is mainly about your imagination... ... about adjusting your thoughts and images to letting go... ... You can do this whenever you want, again and again... ... because whenever feelings of guilt might plague you or just arise... ... you focus on your breathing and imagine feelings of guilt like heavy stones crumbling to dust before your eyes... ... and immediately you will feel the relief inside you... ... just like today... ... exactly like today...

Hypnosis 6

Goal Setting and Preparation

You know the feelings of guilt that have long burdened you... ... You have tried to let them go... ... have told yourself that you have taken on too much... ... that you cannot change the past, whether you acted guiltily or just took on guilt and responsibility for someone else... ... Your mind knows it is time to let go of the old feelings of guilt... ... but so far, it has not succeeded in feeling... ... But today you want to take this step... ... want to free yourself in feeling... ... You succeed when you can understand why you have held on to the feeling of guilt for so long... ... today it is possible, and maybe you are already wondering how it can succeed today... ... So let's begin so you can experience it...

Setting Up the Place of Encounter

Imagine you are standing in front of an old house... ... it is a stately, large house, and you are standing directly in front of it... ... It is a house of encounter where you can meet a special guest today... ... in your imagination and in your feeling... ... You open the door and enter inside... ... In the cloakroom in the entrance area, you put down all burdens... ... all bags and items you might be carrying... ... You empty your pockets and take off your shoes... ... and then you walk through a corridor... ... It leads directly to a room that is open... ... You enter... ... in the room, there are only two chairs facing each other, nothing else... ... You sit down on one of the chairs...

Encounter with the Inner Helper

You close your eyes in this room and think about the feeling of guilt again... ... You remember trying to let it go, but somehow you still held on to it... ... Maybe it felt like the guilt was holding you... ... or something inside you was holding on to it... ... You wonder what that was and is... ... and with this question in your thoughts, you open your eyes in the old house and see an old man/woman (please adjust to the client's gender) sitting opposite you on the chair... ... The person introduces themselves as your inner helper... ... a part of you that comes here today to help you... ... At this moment, you connect internally with yourself... ... It happens automatically because you are always connected with yourself... ... but now, in this trance... ... in the imagination of being in a house, in a room... ... with two chairs, sitting opposite yourself, you also connect in your attention and mindfulness... ... focus on yourself, sitting opposite yourself... ... can look at this old and experienced part of yourself...

Confrontation and Clarification

And once again, you ask why this part of you, now sitting opposite you, has held on to guilt for so long... ... Look into the inner helper's face... ... his/her lips move because he/she is now answering you... ... Listen to the answer or feel it deep inside... ... [Please allow about 30 seconds] ... ... Just accept what the person tells you because it is a message from within... ... from your deep inner self, from your inner center... ... but even if you couldn't hear or feel the answer yet, it is already here... ... it lies in your feeling and can show itself very soon... ... your inner helper is here to really help you... ... with answers, but also with actions... ... so you give the helping person, this helping part of yourself, the task of taking the feelings of guilt away now because you no longer need them... ... You know or feel deep inside why you held on to them for so long... ... why this feeling was still there... ... but now it can go because you don't need it anymore... ... You have long since moved on... ... have developed, resolved or understood old questions and ambiguities... ... or recognized that you cannot change the past and that feelings of guilt cannot do that either... ... Your helper leaves the room... ... they take the feelings of guilt with them because they belong to them... ... This part of your personality has held the feeling of guilt for so long... ... this part lets it go now to help you be free again... ... The person who helped you leaves the room with all the old and outdated feelings of guilt...

Consolidation (Post-Hypnotic Suggestion)

You think about the encounter with your inner helper and trust that he/she will always take away and let go of feelings of guilt deep inside because this helper is a part of you... ... the part that used to hold on and now can let go... ... who else would do that but this part... ... He/She lets go now... ... and whenever old thoughts of guilt could arise again, even before they can become strong, this part of you starts to move to let go of the guilt for you... ... always let go... ... until the feelings of guilt are forgotten...

Hypnosis 7

Goal Setting and Preparation

Today you want to let go of old feelings of guilt that you know do not truly belong to you... ... You have recognized that you are not guilty and that it is high time to build up a good and free feeling again... ... Somehow the old feeling of guilt stayed with you... ... You tried to let it go, but old thoughts and old patterns of responsibility led to you not getting rid of it yet... ... today it should be different... ... Your body feeling can help you with this... ... maybe you know that all feelings we have are also stored in the body... ... You know the gut feeling that often shows you even before the thoughts that something is not right... ... Your gut feeling can also indicate when you feel guilty... ... and often you have felt guilty even though you had no responsibility for things that happened... ... or for omissions that were not yours... ... Guilt is like a burden inside...

Somato-Emotional Change

But your body feeling can help you... ... can help you have and recognize other feelings... ... feelings that are also there... ... but often it is difficult to really feel what the body signals... ... and so you may not have noticed that your body has long signaled that the old feelings of guilt are gone... ... that it has let them go... ... because the body does not err... ... but the mind sometimes holds on to its own beliefs... ... Now concentrate on the feeling of your body... ... feel your gut clearly... ... I will now place my hand on your stomach... ... [Place your hand loosely on the client's solar plexus] ... ... You feel my hand on your stomach; it helps you perceive your body feeling better... ... When you now think about your feelings of guilt and remember how often they bothered you, burdened you, and weighed down your thoughts... ... [Apply slightly more pressure with the hand slowly] ... ... then you suddenly feel my hand as a burden on your body, even though it is just lying there... ... It seems heavier to you because your body shows what you deeply feel inside... ... and guilt feels heavy... ... like a heavy burden... ... and maybe you have often felt this burden physically... ... as pressure in the gut feeling... ... as aching shoulders or as back pain... ... and like a heavy hand on the stomach, which is actually so light... ... Stay in the memory a little longer to clearly feel that your body shows what you think... ... that your body shows what you feel... ... because then you can also more easily feel how change occurs... ... how you become light again inside... ... It works, and you can do it... ... You can let go of feelings of guilt, just like that, because you want to... ... It was only your thoughts that doubted... ... You were not sure if it had succeeded, and then the feeling of guilt could return... ... But today you learn to trust your body feeling and feel that you let go of feelings of guilt... ... You don't need them anymore... ... They only stand in your way and have long since served their purpose...

... ... So now concentrate on the thought of letting go of guilt that you no longer need and do not want... ... You let go of it internally now... ... To do this, you only need the thought that you want to let it go and some concentration and attention that you direct to your body feeling... ... to where my hand lies... ... because your gut feeling will slowly show you that you are letting go of the old guilt... ... because the pressure subsides... ... [Now slowly reduce the pressure with your hand, but keep the hand on the stomach to maintain contact] ... ... You let go of feelings of guilt and the pressure escapes... ... You now let go of all feelings of guilt, and the pressure escapes... ... It feels lighter... ... my hand feels light on your stomach, just like the whole time... ... but now... ... step by step, it also feels lighter... ... because your body recognizes the inner lightness and shows it in feeling... ... so tensions in the shoulders disappear... ... so back pain dissolves and disappears... ... so you become light inside... ... deeply light inside... ... because you can let go of feelings of guilt, and you let them go... ... You have often let them go, only your thoughts could doubt... ... So you often didn't know if you still had guilt or a bad conscience... ... felt this uncertainty and mistook it for guilt... ... but today it is different... ... today you let go of guilt thoughts and feel the lightness in the gut feeling... ... because you become light inside... ... ... Now I take my hand away because you now have a good feeling for your body, can feel load and relief yourself... ... [Remove hand and do not place it on the body again!] ... ... Now remember your former feeling of guilt... ... Feel that the thought of guilt creates a burden in your gut feeling... ... Remember the former guilt and feel the burden in your gut... ... It is only memory... ... and now think that you have let go of the guilt and let it go again... ... and feel the lighter feeling in your gut... ... You can feel it... ... You become light inside... ... and feel the relief in your gut...

Consolidation (Post-Hypnotic Suggestion)

You succeed every day... ... because every day you can lie down quietly for a few minutes and feel your body consciously and feel what you feel... ... then you can remember... ... difficult phases and feelings or even beautiful ones and thus feel how your body feeling changes at that moment... ... and in letting go of thoughts and memories, your body feeling changes again... ... so your body can always help you recognize what you really feel... ... so you can feel in the body that you have overcome painful or burdensome feelings in your deep emotions... ... that you have let them go because you no longer need them... ... because they have long since served their purpose...

Hypnosis 8

Ideomotorics refers to the phenomenon that our body follows our feelings and thoughts with movements. In everyday life, this following shows as posture, muscle tension, and movement patterns of a person, which naturally change with mood and thoughts. In trance, ideomotor signals can be used to get information that the client cannot actively share. The subconscious can, for example, answer questions with an agreed finger signal. Of course, ideomotor reactions can also be used suggestively, for example in arm levitations and catalepsies. An approach I also use in the following text strengthens trust in hypnosis and in one's ability to change and thus promotes therapy.

Goal Setting and Preparation

You want to let go of the tormenting feelings of guilt... ... You want to free yourself from a bad conscience and the thoughts that you are always responsible... ... You have often tried, but then the feelings of guilt came back because you could not really imagine that they would get smaller and disappear... ... because you could not quite believe that they would indeed get smaller and disappear... ... Today you can get special help, help from your subconscious... ... maybe you are wondering how exactly that can work... ... how exactly it can work... ... so this hypnosis becomes an exciting journey for you... ... We can ask your subconscious if it can do that... ... we can ask it to show you that it can let go of the feelings of guilt deep inside... ... because it indeed can... ... So let's go...

Establishing Catalepsy

Now concentrate on your wish to let go of the feelings of guilt... ... Imagine how nice it would be if it were already done... ... how good it can feel to be completely free of feelings of guilt... ... Place your hands loosely beside your body... ... with the palms facing up... ... Keep the hands very loose, and above all... ... Don't help me... ... Everything that needs to be done is done by your subconscious... ... You have tried actively again and again to let go of feelings of guilt, but it has not yet succeeded... ... Now do nothing... ... Take in my words and don't help me with it... ... Your subconscious can and will act for you... ... Your deep inner self can and will let go of the feelings of guilt for you... ... Formulate this wish, your goal in your thoughts, and tell your subconscious... ... Let go of my feelings of guilt now... ... and your subconscious will let go of all the old feelings of guilt and the bad conscience... ... because all feelings of guilt are stored in your body and flow into your open hands... ... all feelings of guilt dissolve and flow now into your open hands, which may feel heavy because of it... ... That is perfectly fine because you will soon let go of the feelings of guilt... ... All feelings of guilt flow into the hands... ... right and left... ... and make the hands heavy... ... All feelings of guilt flow into the hands... ... right and left... ... and make the hands heavy... ... very good... ... You are doing it exactly right... ... Your hands are getting heavier and more immobile... ... heavy as lead and completely immobile because they now hold this guilt alone... ... Only your hands hold the guilt... ... the hands are getting heavier... ... because they hold the heavy feelings of guilt... ... and that is all good because now the change can begin...

Ideomotor Task

Your subconscious now ends the feelings of guilt, lets them go at last... ... Your subconscious can now let go of the feelings of guilt... ... and thus your hands become lighter and start to turn... ... your hands now become lighter and lighter because you are letting go of the feelings of guilt... ... You recognize this by the fact that your hands turn because you empty the full hands... ... The more feelings of guilt your subconscious lets go of, the more your hands turn, becoming lighter and lighter... ... Your hands become lighter and turn... ... your hands become lighter and turn... ... [Wait for the complete turning of both hands!] ...

[Try to be patient if it takes a while for the hands to turn. Ideomotor signals are reliable signs, similar to kinesiology muscle tests. Here we work with a mixture of suggestive encouragement and ideomotor communication. If you repeatedly say... Your hands turn... it has a suggestive effect, and the ideomotor reaction follows. By implying that this is associated with letting go of the feelings of guilt, a coupling occurs in the subconscious. The subconscious confirms the letting go at the same time. If letting go were not possible, it would not make sense to turn the hands. If the turning only occurs due to the suggestion, it is still proof to the mind of letting go, as it was "agreed" upon. If the mind is convinced, the goal is almost achieved. Try it out. The effect may surprise you.]

Resolving Catalepsy

Your subconscious has let go of the feelings of guilt and made your hands light again... ... with this, you have achieved a lot and will feel this new freedom in your everyday life... ... Your hands are now light and movable again because they are open to new things... ... Your subconscious gives you back full control of your hands, which may feel good... ... You can check it... ... Move your hands and fingers and check that your hands are completely under your conscious control...

[Always make sure that the client has full conscious control of their hands and fingers again and can move them. Let them actively try it. If it doesn't work, help with further suggestions... Your hands and fingers relax completely, are very loose. Very, very loose are your hands and fingers... You can move them...]

Consolidation (Post-Hypnotic Suggestion)

Your subconscious could free you from feelings of guilt today... ... by turning your hands... ... and you can do it too... ... You can repeat it very simply in your waking life... ... If you ever have the thought that you might have a feeling of guilt you don't want at all... ... or if a spark of a bad conscience comes up, then just briefly close both hands into a fist and open them again in a waking state... ... it immediately reminds your deep inner self of letting go of the feelings of guilt... ... just like today... ... just as simple and just as fast as today...

Hypnosis 9

Preparation

You are here today for a specific reason... ... have often and repeatedly dealt with difficulties and problems... ... have tried to address your issues and do something so that you can feel better... ... have tried to let go of old feelings of guilt and a bad conscience because these feelings no longer help you... ... They only block you so far, and even working on them is often like a brake... ... Today it can be different because today you don't need to deal with it at all... ... Today you can just let everything happen and maybe be surprised how well it works and how much it can help you... ... So allow yourself to do nothing now...

Presupposition

Doing nothing means just following a visual image... ... that you imagine a very simple picture that I will present to you in a few moments... ... Then you don't have to do anything else, just imagine the picture, and that happens quite automatically when I talk about it... ... The better you succeed in just looking at this picture, the faster you reach your goal... ... or more precisely: the goal reaches you...

Current State and Goal Setting

So far, it has been like this... ... You often feel guilty, often have a bad conscience... ... and from now on it should be like this...

Complete freedom from feelings of guilt, inner harmony with your thinking and actions

... [Feel free to place your palm on the client's solar plexus when stating the goal and then pull it away again. This is not necessary, but it helps a lot because the goal is thus "anchored." Of course, you can also integrate energetic techniques into the hypnosis. Make sure not to repeat the goal.] ...

Building the Energy-Balancing Framework

Now direct your attention to your breath and feel how your breath flows in and out... ... in and out... ... [in the client's breathing rhythm] ... ... in and out... ... and now continue to pay attention to the flow of your breath and imagine that there is a small golden light sphere inside your body... ... in your solar plexus... ... a small sphere of pure golden light... ... pleasantly warm and beautiful... ... Focus completely on the image of this light sphere and let it grow a little bigger with each breath... ... with each breath, the light sphere grows a little bigger... ... Let your breath flow calmly... ... breathe in and out calmly... ... and with each breath, the golden light sphere in your inner center becomes a little bigger... ... and bigger... ... [in the client's breathing rhythm] ... ... and bigger... ... very good... ... The light sphere is now as big as a ball and continues to expand... ... Its edge gently extends outside your body... ... and the sphere of golden light gets bigger and bigger... ... and bigger... ... and now surrounds your body from the outside... ... in a few breaths, your whole body will be surrounded by this light shell... ... just a few more breaths, and it will be... ... Your body is completely surrounded by this light sphere... ... You are in the middle of the golden sphere, which continues to grow and grow... ... With each breath, it expands further... ... until it surrounds the building you are in and continues to grow... ... The bigger the light sphere gets, the faster it grows... ... and soon it reaches above the clouds... ... and encompasses the entire earth, becoming the atmosphere of the earth... ... a golden atmosphere that reaches into space... ... a huge sphere of golden light surrounds the entire earth... ... and in the middle of the light sphere, you are breathing calmly... ... You are the center of the light sphere... ... At this moment, you are the center of the world... ... the center of the world...

... ... Continue to breathe calmly and evenly... ... calmly and evenly... ... and imagine how the light sphere gets smaller with each exhale... ... smaller with each breath out... ... The sphere gets smaller... ... [in the client's breathing rhythm] ... ... and smaller... ... [in the client's breathing rhythm] ... ... and smaller... ... It returns to the clouds and brings the full power of the universe to its center... ... to the center where you are... ... The light sphere returns to you... ... gets smaller and brings the power of the earth with it... ... The sphere surrounds the building we are in... ... comes through the walls and is here in the room, surrounding your entire body, which is always in the middle of the golden light sphere... ... and finally, it is so small again that it is entirely inside your body and remains there as a powerful sphere of golden light... ... in your inner center... ... in your solar plexus...

Dissolving the Energetic Framework

Now let your thoughts go back and forth... ... No thought is important now... ... There is nothing more to do because everything has already happened... ... everything is already done... ... Let go of the image of the light sphere because it will stay with you as a feeling... ... Feel the connection to your body and the surface...

Hypnosis 10

Arriving in the Land of Dreams

In our nightly dreams, there are no limits; everything we can imagine can happen there... ... there are no laws of nature, no boundaries, no logic, and no mind... ... it is our feelings that create all the images and scenes of the dreams... ... and dreams are always images and scenes about ourselves... ... Our dreams tell us about ourselves, even if we think we are dreaming about other people... ... In our daydreams, it is exactly the same... ... they too run without limits... ... daydreams also allow us the same insight into our deep inner self... ... into the realm of the unconscious and feelings... ... because our daydreams are shaped by our longings and desires... ... by fantasy and creativity... ... They are always our feelings that create our dreams... ... You find every single dream in this special land inside you... ... in the land of dreams... ... Your breath carries you there... ... It blows your thoughts like a gentle wind into the land of dreams... ... You are already there... ...

are deep in the land of unlimited possibilities inside you... ... You are in the land of dreams...

Confrontation, Clarification, Creative Reorientation

You stand by a small river in the forest... ... The river winds through the forest, you can hear the sound of flowing water... ... and on the riverbank, you start walking... ... go against the current, upstream... ... your path leads you through the bright forest... ... You walk on a narrow path that looks as if no one has ever been here before... ... there are no footprints here yet... ... and that is really good because it is your new path... ... and on a truly new path, there can be no footprints yet... ... The land of dreams is your land... ... the land of your emotions and moods... ... here there can always only be your footprints... ... and so your tracks now first meet this path... ... You follow the river's path, and the sound of flowing water becomes more intense and stronger... ... Then you see through the trees a small waterfall where your path leads... ... You approach the waterfall... ... and when you reach the waterfall, you stop and watch the water stream down... ... It is crystal clear... ... very pure... ... and the sunlight sparkles and glitters on the streaming water... ... You think about the feelings of guilt inside you... ... You look dreamily at the stream of water, and situations where you felt guilty come to mind... ... or events that happened so quickly that you didn't have time to think and weigh things... ... maybe acted spontaneously or in anger... ... maybe in euphoria and exuberance... ... and later you regretted it, felt you did something wrong... ... asked yourself if your actions were right... ... or permissible... ... or just... ... You look at the images of the memory again... ... let them rise in your thoughts again or just wait because they show themselves at the waterfall... ... You look at the sparkling water... ... as if you could see through the waterfall... ... and in this deep dreamy gaze, images rise again... ... maybe memories you haven't had for a long time... ... possibly events you thought didn't burden you so far... ... but now you remember... ... recognize that there were also some deep-seated feelings of guilt that gave you a bad conscience... ... or others that amplified conscious thoughts of guilt without you noticing... ... often, it is not just the obvious and big events that create our feelings of guilt, but many small events where we have been strict with ourselves... ... as strict as you were with yourself... ... because you intended to always be a good person and harm as few people as possible... ... not to cause anyone a disadvantage... ... but that is not always possible... ... People make mistakes... ... but forgiving others is usually easier for you than forgiving yourself... ... You remember that now... ... and you also remember and can see in images that you have blamed yourself for many things without even having truly guilty omissions... ... Let the images just be there because it is important to see them once more... ... because today you can let them go... ... not only let go of the images but the feelings of guilt... ... because images remain as memories in you, help you develop further, not to experience and do the same thing over and over... ... but the feelings of guilt can go today... ... but maybe you don't see any images deep inside you... ... can't recognize them now... ... if that's the case, that's perfectly fine because all your memories are stored in you... ... in images and in feelings, and therefore all important feelings are here... ... especially the feeling of guilt... ... that you can let go of today... ... You step into the river... ... step into the water, which is only knee-deep... ... You can stand well in it, very stable because nothing can happen to you in the land of dreams... ... You walk through the water to the waterfall...

... and you stand in the stream of water... ... You feel the water on your body... ... It feels pleasant and warm and becomes a deep inner purification... ... The land of dreams is a land deep inside you, so nothing happens here just like that... ... everything has a meaning... ... and this waterfall serves for inner purification... ... it washes the old feelings of guilt away from you... ... You look at your skin and can see that it becomes clean... ... the more water runs down on you, the brighter your skin shines... ... your whole body shines...

Mindfulness and Self-Loyalty

The old feelings of guilt are taken by the river and preserved as memories... ... but everything becomes light inside you, you are freed from this old feeling... ... everything remains, but everything in its place... ... nothing is erased, but everything finds its place... ... Guilt in the place of memory... ... and where it was before, the feeling of freedom arises... ... This feeling was always there too, but until now in the wrong place... ... now everything is sorted... ... Guilt is memory... ... Freedom is conscious... ... In thoughts, let the water continue to flow and think about the fact that the land of dreams is deep inside you... ... it was always there... ... I only tell you about it...

Distribution, publication, and copying in any form are prohibited and subject to damages.

Overview of All Titles in the Series "Ten Hypnoses"

Volume 1: Smoking Cessation
Volume 2: Anxiety and Restlessness
Volume 3: Burnout
Volume 4: Reducing Overweight
Volume 5: Coping with the Past
Volume 6: Suicidal Thoughts and Attempts
Volume 7: Psycho-Oncology
Volume 8: Obsessions and Tics
Volume 9: Self-Confidence and Decision-Making
Volume 10: Grief Work
Volume 11: Psychosomatics
Volume 12: Chronic Pain
Volume 13: Depressive Thoughts
Volume 14: Panic Attacks
Volume 15: Domestic Violence, Victim Support
Volume 16: Post-Traumatic Stress
Volume 17: Exam Anxiety and Stage Fright
Volume 18: Anti-Violence Training, Offender Support
Volume 19: Addiction Tendencies
Volume 20: Social Phobia and Fear of Contact
Volume 21: Nail Biting
Volume 22: Self-Awareness and Self-Love
Volume 23: Teeth Grinding and Night Clenching
Volume 24: Feelings of Guilt
Volume 25: Fear in Crowds
Volume 26: Fear of Flying, Aviophobia
Volume 27: Fear in Enclosed Spaces, Claustrophobia
Volume 28: Tinnitus, Ear Noises
Volume 29: Fear of Heights
Volume 30: Neurodermatitis

Copying, publishing, and sharing with third parties are only permitted with the written consent of the author. Please observe the notes on copyright and usage.

Volume 31: Finding Inner Balance
Volume 32: Overcoming Loneliness
Volume 33: Fear of Illness, Hypochondria
Volume 34: Anticipatory Anxiety, Fear of Fear
Volume 35: Jealousy in Relationships
Volume 36: Driving Anxiety
Volume 37: New Start after Separation
Volume 38: Fear of Injections
Volume 39: Heart Anxiety Neurosis
Volume 40: Overcoming Resentment and Anger
Volume 41: Resolving Blockages and Positive Thinking
Volume 42: Stress Reduction, Stress Management
Volume 43: Body Relaxation
Volume 44: Deep Relaxation
Volume 45: Fear of the Dark
Volume 46: Falling Asleep and Staying Asleep
Volume 47: Compulsive Buying
Volume 48: Restless Legs Syndrome
Volume 49: Bulimia
Volume 50: Anorexia
Volume 51: Overcoming Nightmares
Volume 52: Imagined Deformity
Volume 53: Overcoming Distrust, Finding Trust
Volume 54: Processing Failures
Volume 55: Humiliation, Emotional Hurt
Volume 56: Distressing Compassion, Vicarious Suffering
Volume 57: Self-Forgiveness
Volume 58: Self-Awareness, Self-Confidence
Volume 59: Saying No
Volume 60: Assertiveness
Volume 61: Setting Boundaries and Self-Assertion
Volume 62: Decision-Making Ability

Volume 63: Success Orientation
Volume 64: Ruminating, Circular Thinking
Volume 65: Accepting Pregnancy
Volume 66: Birth Preparation
Volume 67: Spiritual Opening
Volume 68: Joy of Life and Inner Lightness
Volume 69: Patience and Inner Peace
Volume 70: Fibromyalgia and Rheumatism
Volume 71: Irritable Bowel Syndrome, Crohn's Disease
Volume 72: Fear of Nausea, Emetophobia
Volume 73: Stuttering and Cluttering, Speech Flow Disorders
Volume 74: Concentration and Knowledge Anchoring
Volume 75: Vitality and Spontaneity
Volume 76: Searching for Meaning and Finding Goals
Volume 77: Life Crises, Life Events
Volume 78: Workaholism, Goal Obsession
Volume 79: Helper Syndrome, Helpless Helpers
Volume 80: Medication Abuse
Volume 81: Gambling Addiction
Volume 82: Internet Addiction, Smartphone Addiction
Volume 83: Hoarding Disorder, Compulsive Collecting
Volume 84: Conspiracy Thoughts, Overvalued Ideas
Volume 85: Fear of Operations and Treatments
Volume 86: Fear of Aging
Volume 87: Travel Anxiety
Volume 88: Anxiety When Urinating, Paruresis
Volume 89: Fear of Intimacy and Togetherness
Volume 90: Fear of Blushing
Volume 91: Coming Out in Homosexuality
Volume 92: Charisma Training
Volume 93: Migraines and Chronic Headaches
Volume 94: Overcoming Allergies, Bronchial Asthma

Volume 95: Normalizing Blood Pressure
Volume 96: Compulsive Perfectionism
Volume 97: Sports Hypnosis, Motivation
Volume 98: Sports Hypnosis, Performance Enhancement
Volume 99: Determination and Focus
Volume 100: Encountering the Inner Child
Volume 101: Cravings, Binge Eating
Volume 102: Stimulating Metabolism
Volume 103: Bipolar Mood Swings
Volume 104: Borderline, Identity Crises
Volume 105: Hypomania, Euphoria, Mania
Volume 106: Restlessness, Agitation
Volume 107: Nervous Breakdown
Volume 108: Adjustment Disorders
Volume 109: Self-Alienation, Depersonalization
Volume 110: Ending Self-Pity
Volume 111: Primary Gain of Illness
Volume 112: Secondary Gain of Illness
Volume 113: Bullying, Victim Support
Volume 114: Letting Go of Envy and Jealousy
Volume 115: Fear of Spiders, Arachnophobia
Volume 116: Fear of Dogs or Cats
Volume 117: Fear of Strangers, Xenophobia
Volume 118: Excessive Worries, Generalized Anxiety
Volume 119: Strengthening Sense of Responsibility
Volume 120: Unrequited Love, Heartache
Volume 121: Work-Life Balance
Volume 122: Letting Go of Unattainable Goals
Volume 123: Allowing and Accepting Help
Volume 124: Letting Go of Adult Children
Volume 125: Tourette Syndrome
Volume 126: Life Changes and New Starts

Volume 127: Accepting Life in a Wheelchair
Volume 128: Understanding and Overcoming Homesickness
Volume 129: Understanding and Overcoming Wanderlust
Volume 130: Dizziness, Meniere's Disease
Volume 131: Overcoming Aggression
Volume 132: Cutting and Self-Harm
Volume 133: Hair Pulling, Trichotillomania
Volume 134: Postpartum Depression
Volume 135: For Relatives of Dementia Patients
Volume 136: Self-Harm, Artificial Disorders
Volume 137: Activating Self-Healing Powers
Volume 138: Preventing Depression Relapse
Volume 139: Reactive Psychoses, Follow-Up
Volume 140: Obsessive Thoughts and Impulses
Volume 141: Compulsive Checking
Volume 142: Compulsive Counting, Symmetry Obsession
Volume 143: Compulsive Washing, Cleanliness Obsession
Volume 144: Compulsive Questioning
Volume 145: Dissociative Paralysis
Volume 146: Phantom Pain
Volume 147: Overcoming Complaining
Volume 148: Hay Fever, Pollen Allergy
Volume 149: Sexual Abuse, Victim Support
Volume 150: Standing Strong Against Sexism, #metoo
Volume 151: Binge Eating
Volume 152: Overcoming Thoughts of Revenge
Volume 153: Detachment from the Aggressor, Stockholm Syndrome
Volume 154: Courage to Separate
Volume 155: Chronic Fatigue, Exhaustion
Volume 156: Fear of the Future, Existential Anxiety
Volume 157: Excessive Worry About Children
Volume 158: Fear of Failure

Volume 159: Ending Distrust and Control
Volume 160: Dejection, Dysphoria
Volume 161: Boreout, Chronic Boredom
Volume 162: Bipolar Disorders, Relapse Prevention
Volume 163: Mania, Relapse Prevention
Volume 164: Nihilism, Feelings of Worthlessness
Volume 165: Thumb Sucking
Volume 166: Being Brave
Volume 167: Being Proud
Volume 168: Overcoming Shyness
Volume 169: Being Able to Delegate Responsibility
Volume 170: Being Able to Show Emotions
Volume 171: Letting Go of Guilt, Victim Support
Volume 172: Processing Guilt, Offender Support
Volume 173: Mood Swings, Cyclothymia
Volume 174: Lack of Drive, Vital Sadness
Volume 175: Hearing Voices with Reality Reference
Volume 176: Confident Communication
Volume 177: Standing Up for Oneself
Volume 178: Taking New Paths
Volume 179: Confident Job Application
Volume 180: No Longer Being Taken Advantage Of
Volume 181: End of Submissiveness
Volume 182: Depressive Numbness
Volume 183: Mood Drops, Affective Incontinence
Volume 184: Mood Instability
Volume 185: Somatoform Disorders
Volume 186: Stomach Ulcer, Psychosomatic
Volume 187: Accepting Amputation
Volume 188: Overcoming and Letting Go of Hatred
Volume 189: Ending Accusations
Volume 190: Allowing Tears, Being Able to Cry

Volume 191: Finding and Sorting Repressed Feelings
Volume 192: Somatoform Pain
Volume 193: Living Autonomously
Volume 194: Anhedonia, Joylessness
Volume 195: Persistent Sadness
Volume 196: Obesity, Food Addiction
Volume 197: Parents of Abused Children
Volume 198: Letting Go and Letting Be
Volume 199: Childhood Sexual Abuse
Volume 200: Fear of Loss

www.ingramcontent.com/pod-product-compliance
Lightning Source LLC
Chambersburg PA
CBHW030501220526
45464CB00006B/2603